Inner Journey:
The Enemy Within

Inner Journey:
The Enemy Within

Victoria Ann Heirston

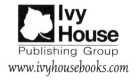

Ivy House
Publishing Group
www.ivyhousebooks.com

PUBLISHED BY IVY HOUSE PUBLISHING GROUP
5122 Bur Oak Circle, Raleigh, NC 27612
United States of America
919-782-0281

ISBN: 1-57197-343-5
Library of Congress Control Number: 2002112994

Printed in the United States of America

Acknowledgments

I, hereby, give heartfelt gratitude to all those at Child and Family Services, Broadway, Amityville, New York, for all their kindness and especially a hearty thanks to Mr. Richard Gordon, Dr. Dormesy and Susan. I'll never forget you and what you have done for me and my life. Hope all your wishes come true.

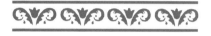

Book I–Chapter One

This is the story of a long journey—one that began many years ago. People very often have trials and tribulations in life that can be attributed to dysfunctional families, health issues, abandonment or abuse. This is not the story I am going to tell.

I was born in Brooklyn, New York, to Viola and Ethan Gainer. Both were from different parts of the South. Both had lived similar family lives. My mother was from Richmond, Virginia and my father was from Portsmouth, Virginia. Both were from middle-class families. They were not children of slaves, but were children of families who had struggled for existence.

My mother's family was extremely fair-skinned. They were hardworking, middle-class people. I was told that my great-grandfather was a notable photographer in the South, with a reputation for very fine work. While I do not know much about him, I have heard some fascinating stories about his work. My grandfather, on the other hand, was employed with the Baltimore and Ohio (B&O) Railroad as a chef, where he met my grandmother and, after a respectable courtship, was married to her. I remember the stories I was told about the wonderful dishes he would bring home, the desserts, fruits, nuts and especially the ice cream that would come home with him after his shift was completed every night. They married and moved to Bayonne, New Jersey, where they started their lives together and raised four children. They later moved to Brooklyn, New York, where my mother met my father. It was in Brooklyn where my parents were married and started their life together.

My father's family came from rural Portsmouth. My father was the son of a black Baptist preacher who did not live long enough to see my father grow up. He died before my father was eight years old. After the death of her husband, Sister Annie Gainer remarried a man that I came to know as my grandfather. His name was Isaac Harrels. He and Annie, I loved so much. I remember summers with them while my parents traveled. I would stay with them all summer. He made me a swing, hung from a very old oak tree that stood in the far corner of the yard. I had chicks that I loved until I lost them in the creek that ran behind the little house on Gosport Road. Brushing my grandmother's long, brown hair remains a pleasant memory for me. I recall long hot days sitting and rocking on the front porch, saying hellos to everyone who passed. These are the memories I will never forget.

I was born on February 14, 1940, a day that my mother later reported was the worst day, weather-wise, of her life. It rained, snowed and was colder than it had ever been before in her memory. My dad, a postal employee, made his way to the hospital on this horrendous Wednesday to see his new baby girl who had been born that morning.

Dad was surprised to see me, so small (only 6 lbs., 7 oz.), blue-eyed and fair skinned. I was the spitting image of his mother, not my father who was dark in color with dark hair and dark eyes. My mother, on the other hand, was very fair-skinned with black hair and dark eyes. But, happily, I took after my father's mother with light hair, eyes and fair skin. My mother's mother was not delighted with the fact that I made her a grandmother. Oh, of course, she came once to see me, but I was not the light of her life. Somehow, I knew that at an early age. My parents only wanted one child, believing that their income and lifestyle would only permit one child. I was not spoiled in any way, but we did live a nice life. My mom and dad were selfishly connected with each other and there were times that I felt I did not belong. I felt isolated and invisible.

My days at Suffolk Psychiatric were bleak. How I got there, I am not sure. I remember my regular weekly visit with Dr. Jiminez, a slight, wiry man, in his early forties, with a receding hairline and a soft manner. He was waiting for me at his office door when I arrived at the Office of Mental Health in Suffolk County that cloudy day in early September. His voice was soft; I had difficulty understanding him from the first time we met. I wondered to myself, *How will I ever get well when I cannot understand what he is saying to me?* English was not his native language and he spoke it with a thick accent.

He invited me into his simply furnished office and asked me to have a seat, which I promptly did. During that particular weekly appointment, I sat in the cold, bare office confessing my heart out to a doctor who could barely speak English and one I did not understand. But, there I sat, begging for help, agonizing over questions he asked, trying to recall events that might have led to my present condition. I felt myself losing control. I began screaming hysterically for him to help me. I couldn't stay this way any longer. I was sinking and there was no one to save me from this quicksand I was succumbing to, no one to give me relief from this terrible fear, this awesome anxiety. I felt deadness slowly enveloping me. "Oh, please help me," I begged, "please help me."

Standing in the waiting room of Suffolk Psychiatric Hospital, the one and only question I remember being asked was, "Are you voluntarily signing yourself into this institution?" I immediately answered, "Yes." I was so glad to be there. Later I learned that Dr. Jiminez had called my mom and she drove me there through the bleakness of that dark, rainy night. I felt so sorry for her. She looked so pained, so lost and sad, as if asking the question, *Is this really happening to us? How did it happen, why is it happening?* For me, I had reached a safe haven, but for her it was going to be difficult. Therefore, my sadness was more for her than for myself.

The interior of the building was dingy and drab. The room, a nondescript gray, desperately in need of paint. I said good-bye to my mother, watching as she walked away, escorted by hospital personnel. With a tear in my eye, I was left with my new associates in my new home. I was slightly frightened and uneasy, but I accepted everything in stride. There was a certain peace I had not felt for a very long time, if ever. The matron took me into a room where six to eight cots lined the wall, leaving only a small aisle down the center in which to walk. I was introduced to some women, their names I have since forgotten. I hardly remember meeting them. I was given a shot of medication and allowed to slip out of my street clothes and into some sleepwear provided by the hospital. I remember no more of that night, only that it was the beginning of my hope for recovery.

Days at the hospital were endless and the nights were longer. I went from day to night in a fog, starting with breakfast and ending with television at night. It was summertime and the weather was oppressive. The grounds were hot, dry and barren except for the robot-like bodies that occasionally traversed the walkways going from dormitory to dormitory or to the dining hall to eat. There were no schedules, no pressures and no commitments except for the group therapy sessions that had to be attended in the afternoon and at night when it was time to dispense the medication. Visitors were sparse and sometimes appeared on the grounds sitting under the trees or on the benches speaking quietly with the patients they had come to visit.

Remembering those visits is hard, although I know my mother was there and on some occasions brought my daughter, Kelley, with her. We did not say much to each other. I remember long silences in which nothing was said. We sat as if we were two strangers sharing a park bench in the heat of the afternoon sun. We did not touch each other's hand, nor were hugs exchanged. There were no discussions about life inside the hospital or what my mom was doing in her daily routine with Kelley. I don't remember these things being discussed; maybe they were and I just do not remember. I do recall the long and uncomfortable silences. My mother was a good person, but not capable of showing the warmth and love that I so desperately needed. Hugs, as a child, were unavailable as were the compliments and affirmations of self-worth and value everyone needs. It was hard on my mom and I certainly understood. A recent widow, left with my three-year-old child to care for and me, her emotionally sick daughter, in a psychiatric hospital for chronic depression, facing the possibility of shock therapy. Could things have been any worse for us? We were generations divided, but brought close through our mutual suffering.

Shock therapy began after recommendations from the staff doctors. Only when my blood pressure became abnormally elevated did they discontinue their course of treatment. My memories are vague and abstract. I can remember the orange juice or other sweet treat given after the therapy was over. There was little conversation, only directions given regarding the administration of the treatment.

After medication, we would meet for group therapy in a large, scantily furnished, dreary room that contained old, used furniture. Sitting opposite our fellow "inmates," we would share parts of our lives with perfect strangers. Some were overly hostile and unfriendly, others were too friendly and still others had to be physically removed to the upper floor to be contained because they would begin to be disruptive. The floor above us, I later learned, was reserved for patients that were severely depressed, psychotic or for other extreme cases.

Days went into weeks and weeks into months. I made very few friends, keeping to myself for the most part, and waited for my mother's visits. I still realized that there was an outside world and I still had a grasp on reality.

I felt a good part of my life departed from me during those long, still days of summer. There was no yesterday, no today and no tomorrow. Everything felt empty, barren as the days moved towards the fall of the year. People disappeared from the grounds; music heard all summer was no more. Visits from the outside world became scarce and the weather became bleak. But, my recovery was slow and steady.

La Familia

Let me now tell you the story of my family. Originating in Virginia in the early 1900s, there was William Farley and Rebecca Lavaliere, who were very much in love. Never had it been seen in those parts two people more in love than William and Rebecca. She was a beautiful Southern belle with hair down to her waist, a tiny figure with dark black eyes and hair. She was something to behold at a very early age and caught the attention of William Farley, a handsome specimen of a man who was so attracted to the lovely Rebecca that he asked the family for her hand in marriage. William Farley was a good catch, not only because of his good looks but he dressed impeccably, appearing quite dapper in his three-piece vested suits, Italian shoes, fancy cars and jewelry. His home was majestic. You see, William Farley was the leading photographer known all over the world for his exceptional work. He was also known to be a runaround, making babies and leaving them and their mothers as fast as he made them. But Rebecca paid no attention to the warning signs and married him anyway. These were my great-grandparents.

William and Rebecca had several daughters: Rebecca, named after her mother, Eva and Victoria. Now Victoria looked just like her mother, a real beauty and personality to go along with it. She was a very popular young lady. The boys continuously sought her out for their attention and she was always very aloof and unavailable, which would tend to drive them crazy. When Victoria met Louis Price, it was disastrous. No one knew him. He was not a homespun Virginian. They were suspicious and skeptical about this man. But Victoria was not at all intimidated. She loved Louis and that was all there was to that. Nothing would stop her from having and marrying him. Now, Louis was a chef, not at a well-known or well-respected restaurant. Rather, Louis was a chef on the Baltimore and Ohio (B&O) Railroad. This meant he was not home each night and that he spent nights away from home, traveling from city to city. But all of this was all right with Rebecca. She knew she loved and wanted to marry Louis, against her family's advice.

After their marriage and before the children arrived, Louis had to tell Victoria that they were going to move to New York for a career advancement and because that was where the money would be, not in the South where wages were quite low and where there was no chance to move ahead. They headed for Bayonne, New Jersey, living there for a few years before moving to Brooklyn, New York, into one of those lovely brownstones that were built on tree-lined streets of that city. Victoria was very lonely so far from her family and familiar surroundings. It took her quite a long time to adjust, but by the time her first child was due, she was feeling better about being so far away. Fordham weighed in at around ten pounds. He looked exactly like Louis with his dark hair and eyes. He was a handful, but grew up to be a very handsome, talented, shy man. Later, he would strum the guitar and everyone would sit around the kitchen table just to hear him play. Viola, like her mother, was quite a beauty. She was tall and fair-skinned with jet-black hair, but also was shy like Ford. When Viola reached sixteen, all the boys were after her; but like her mother she also was aloof to their attentions. Third to be born was Louis, named after his father. Louis was not quite as attractive as his brother and sister, but was socially outgoing and also very talented. He had knowledge of electronics that afforded him a good lifestyle when he grew up, because his talents were so much in demand. Then, there was Constance, the last of the Price children. Constance was sickly and frail but was talented in that she could create. She sketched and painted everything in sight, from fruit bowls to flowers and even teacups from a perfectly set table.

Although the money was not there the way Victoria was used to, she made the best of it. They always had a roof over their heads, plenty of food on the table, music and plenty of laughter. It was a fun house. Victoria and Louis played with their children as if they, too, were kids. This made for a very happy household. But money was always a problem for Victoria. She could not dress as nicely or go to the fancy places she had been privilege to when she lived in the South.

When Ethan Lafayette Gainer first met Viola Price, he knew that she was the woman he was going to marry. He said so. He knew it from the moment he saw her walking down one of those tree-lined streets on that sunny morning in September. "This is the girl I am going to marry," he said to one of his friends as they exchanged a few words and watched Viola as she wandered past them. With a swish of her backside, she turned the corner as if to say, "I know you are watching me, but I am paying no attention to you." That all changed when she was introduced to Ethan that night at a party they both attended. He was very charming and had spent the last two years at the University of Pennsylvania while working with his brother George in the largest black-owned funeral home in that state. Ethan disliked the work so much that he left George and traveled to Brooklyn. He stayed with old friends who lived across the street from the Price family. Ethan and Viola spent long days and nights together. Before very long they married, took an apartment near to her family and a year later on one of February's coldest days, I was born.

My father was born in the rural part of Virginia in a small-framed house on Gosport Road. There was a coal-burning stove in the tiny dining room and a box filled with huge blocks of ice sat in the kitchen. This was his home. His father died when my father was just a little boy. His mother, Annie, had to raise him alone until she met Isaac Harrels. Isaac immediately sought her attention and, even knowing she had a small boy, wanted very much to marry her. She stayed home taking care of Ethan, keeping the wood-stove burning and emptying the icebox several times a day. She loved to spend her time gossiping with the other ladies on the street and in the church that her first husband had founded and preached for many years. When my father was grown, he left his home and moved to Pennsylvania to work with George in the funeral home. But after determining that was not what he wanted to do, he moved to Brooklyn, right across the street from where the Price family lived.

After I was born I spent many happy hours with my grandparents from the time I was three months old. I loved them very much. That was how it all began, with two people from two different worlds meeting not miles from each other, but right across the street, where fate had a hand in bringing them together.

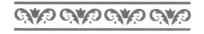

Chapter Two

In my therapy sessions, my earliest recollection was moving at the age of five from Brooklyn to suburban Long Island and a place called South Ozone Park, Jamaica. We moved from the large, three-family brownstone residence where Fat Tony, as he was called, would sit and pick the raisins that had fallen out of his Sunmaid box into the cracks between the steps of the brownstone building. He would search until he would come up with each fallen raisin. The other children in the street were occupied with other play: roller-skating, bicycling and stickball. I remember leaving the neighborhood park, always a favorite with my mother, where green trees had been planted between the blocks of pavement and where the sun always seemed to shine.

Directly across the street lived a craggy, hunched-back old lady that no one knew or visited. The only time the door was ever opened was when she would make her appearance on the littered porch to place another pile of old newspapers. She was strange and scary.

I remember the aroma of spaghetti sauce that filled the stairwell of that three-family walk-up where Mrs. LaPena, the landlady, always seemed to be cooking with garlic, oil and tomato paste. You rarely saw her, but the smell of her sauces attested to her being there. My mom never liked living there.

Mom and I hurried along the concrete streets disappearing down the stairs into the darkness of the New York subway system and on to a waiting train. We both were out of breath when we entered the door and found two seats together. The ride was long and tedious as the train made its way across the tracks, bringing us closer and closer to our destination. My dad had gone ahead with the movers to give directions to our new home. The light, as we slowly ascended from the darkness, was a rude awakening to our sensitive eyes but the sight of our new and different surroundings was a delight to our eyes and hearts. We said very little to each other that day. There was no time for idle chatter, just the anticipation of our arrival at our new home.

The moving van was awaiting our arrival as we stepped off the bus. The sight of the new house was almost too much for my mother as her happiness was very evident. She did not cry, but I could feel the extent of her joy. The view showed middle-class homes dotting tree-lined streets, bright sunshine and clean air. It was a noiseless environment except for the occasional laughter and playfulness of children having a good time. This was so different from the place from which we had come. The smell of honeysuckle permeated the very air as my mother went from room to room opening the windows welcoming the sweet smell, inviting it to come in. Life could not have been better growing up on Long Island in the fifties.

The Glorious Fifties, the decade of promise and light. The Korean War was ending, people were feeling pride and patriotism for their country and new feelings of hope and a positive future were emerging. It was a time of rock 'n' roll, zoot suits, black and white TV, the "Ed Sullivan Show," long and flashy cars, drive-in movies and a general aura of prosperity and wholesomeness. I remember well the long, languid days of summer on Long Island. Most of all, I remember Jones Beach and days spent in the bright, noonday sun and nights spent under the stars at the Marine Theater or the outdoor skating rink. It was a pleasant time for children growing up. Things were simple, life was good. But growing up can be an uneasy emotional time for an adolescent, making the transition from childhood to adulthood, and can be even harder on the parents. Getting to know who you are, where you fit in the social spectrum, peer acceptance, school competitions and physical appearance play havoc with the emerging child entering adulthood.

Marie and Charles Willoughby lived on the same street a few doors away. I looked up to them as if they were icons. They were good-looking, popular, had nice parents and lived in one of the nicest houses in the neighborhood. Marie, the prettiest of all the girls, wore the best clothes, always had money to spend and was popular with the boys. And if that were not enough, she had a doting grandmother who enjoyed seeing her grandchild dressed in the prettiest clothes. Not only did she spend all her money on store-bought clothes, but she also created and designed the most original apparel. No one could afford to dress like Marie no matter how hard the girls tried.

At all the parties it was Marie who made the biggest hit with the boys asking her to be their date. Standing on the sidelines on party night watching as Marie made her way to the dance floor every time, the other wallflowers tried to blend into the woodwork. Each boy would saunter over to the girls as the introduction to the song began. They would make their selection, as if picking a bouquet, leaving the remainder of the girls disappointed, at a loss as to what to do. When the song ended, the dancers would break and each would return to the side of the room from which they had come. The process would begin all over again. I was socially inept, withdrawn and could hardly make conversation, while my friends, Dawn and Fern, flashed around the dance floor like two preening birds, laughing loudly and seducing all the boys to come and dance with them. Fern had extremely long, dark, thick hair and I remember how she would slowly shake her head from side to side smiling sexily while the guys just stood and stared. Dawn, on the other hand, was wild in her dance routines and had the rest of the boys gawking and wishing they could be her partner. It was at these times and in the embarrassment of those moments that I would take to the stairs where I would find the nearest bathroom to escape and lock myself away. There, I could feel safe and secure. I was never there very long before someone would knock on the door, intruding into my space, and I was forced back out into the world I had run from, the world I did not like. I didn't overcome my shyness until much later.

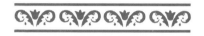

Chapter Three

Meeting the man of my dreams was never a reality. I grew up on fairy tales, soap operas, and, being an only child, I used lots of my imagination and daydreams. I was introspective, escaping the loneliness I felt.

I met Pierre on a day much like any other Saturday. It started when my family did our weekly chores, shopping at the nearby mall, running errands and doing those simple things that must be done at week's end.

A party was being given that night and I was invited to attend. I did not know the host, but received my invitation through my cousin. The crowd was a lot older than I, which made me feel more uncomfortable as the night wore on. Suddenly, out of nowhere, there stood before me this very tall, well-built, nice looking marine in full dress uniform asking me to dance. Inside I was trembling as I felt his warm arms wrap around me. I felt very little confidence in myself in the presence of this very mature stranger. I accepted his invitation to dance, but said very little to him as we made our way around the dance floor. Like Cinderella, I had to run when I was told that my parents had come to pick me up. Although he asked me for my telephone number, the fear of giving it to him made me want to escape.

Six months had passed before he called and then we started dating. Engagement to Pierre came eighteen months after our first meeting. It should have been a joyous time for me, but unfortunately, it was not. I felt compelled to marry this man who seemed to adore me and gave me such a sense of security. My family liked him. I was not in touch with my feelings. I only knew this man loved me, which is something I longed for all my life. My wedding day was a blur of family and friends and good wishes. It rained that September day and everyone said they were showers of blessings.

Our marriage was not consummated that evening in Niagara Falls, Canada, where we were honeymooning, because of a surgical procedure that had to be performed before intimacy could begin. This procedure is known as a hymenectomy, performed to remove the membranous fold which partially or wholly occludes the external vagina. Dr. Vinci would only perform the procedure after the marriage took place. The honeymoon was not what I had dreamed it would be. Pierre was very patient with me during those first days when I was short-tempered, depressed and discouraged. Pierre tried to make everything right with a situation where everything was so wrong. I knew at that time this marriage would not work. There was a missing element and I knew what it was: *love.* I cared for this man, but that was not enough. I did not love him. We spent the next two weeks traveling in Canada enjoying the sights, but I knew that soon the honeymoon would be over.

Playing in my backyard as a child in the fifties, I had the freedom to be anyone I wanted to be and to do anything I wanted to do. I had a vivid imagination and I used it when I thought of marriage and motherhood. I spent many pleasurable hours in that yard fulfilling dreams of one day being a wife and mother. I would dress my favorite doll in one of my romper suits my mother had retrieved from the old clothes box in the attic. She was such a good doll baby. I would feed her and she would wet and I would change her diaper. Making dinner for my make-believe family was always my favorite thing to do with my toy dinnerware, pots and pans, complete with stove and sink. Dinner usually consisted of sweet grapes hand-picked off the arbor next door, grass, weeds and pebbles representing potatoes and vegetables with gravy (that my mother always made), all prepared with great care. My imagination was vivid and I enjoyed my own company, filling many hours that way.

Motherhood, in reality, was a shock and a slight disappointment. I did not relate very well in the beginning. The real world was closing in on me and I did not like what was happening. It was confusing and not at all what I thought it would be. I found myself crumbling under the pressure, torn by my misconceptions and unable to bridge the gap between fantasy and reality. The marriage was slowly deteriorating and there was growing dissension between us. Pierre was controlling and abusive. There were problems—insurmountable problems. I know I have to place some of the responsibility on the Marine Corps where he served over four years, where he learned to fight fearlessly and with courage. But he also learned other lessons in manipulation, terror tactics, abuse and mind control. He had a need to take charge in a dictatorial way, never being wrong or admitting to a fault. Pierre wanted me to be under his control, bending to his wishes and whims. I could not live that way. I began to resent then hate him, but I learned to wait, biding my time before I could eventually leave him.

Oh God, it had been a week! Seven days—and nothing.

I remember thinking as my body lay on the disheveled bed, *Why is this happening to me at this time in my life? Am I sure it has been seven days?* I started counting: Sunday, Monday, Tuesday, Wednesday, Thursday, Friday, Saturday, Sunday. Yes, indeed it had been seven days. My hand began to search between my legs to see if there was any evidence, any sign. But no, there was nothing. *Why is this happening at this time in my life?* I thought. *I don't need this!* That Sunday, while preparing for the beach that hot August morning, I had trouble deciding if I should wear a bathing suit or a pair of shorts, which were a lot safer in case of an accident. I prepared myself, but nothing happened. Maybe exercising, jumping rope or swimming would help. Nothing did. Now it was a week later and still nothing. Many questions ran through my mind. *What am I going to do? I will have to tell Pierre. I can't keep this from him. But what if I don't want this baby? Isn't that my choice?* Considering the weakness in our marriage, that it might not last, how could I consider bringing another life into the mix? We had Kelley, my pride and joy; born to us in 1963, a beautiful dark-haired, dark-eyed baby girl. I did not want another child brought into this already unstable, fragile marriage. I gave this information to my best friend, Dorothy, who wanted to conceive herself, but understood why I did not want another baby. She knew someone. Abortion was illegal in the Sixties. Doctors would not even discuss the issue with you. On my own, I made the appointment with this woman, arriving at her apartment at the scheduled time. Greeting me at the door of her small, darkened apartment I entered the bedroom where I started to slowly remove my clothes. We spoke very little to one another, busying ourselves with the matter at hand. She gave me a pill to relax me and before I realized what was going to happen, my legs were spread apart. She used a sharp instrument, which I later learned was an ordinary coat hanger. There was no pain.

After a few minutes, I got up, lifted my panties, put my clothes on, gave her the money and left. Pierre was home upon my arrival and he was furious with me when he heard the story. I think at that moment that he could have killed me. He was pacing back and forth, hands flailing, his face turning red and I could clearly remember the veins in his neck protruding against his tight skin. He was a large man with a beautiful build, long and lean with wide shoulders, huge upper arms, small waist and long lean legs. His eyes grew larger as he stared at me and I could see the glassiness of his eyes where tears were beginning to form. "How could you do this?" he asked again and again. I felt so full of guilt, fear and disappointment, not with him, but with myself as a human being.

Again, nothing happened. For days, nothing happened. Hot mustard baths, quinine pills, flinging myself down a few steps did nothing. Then, there was that terrible burst of excruciating pain that leveled me and led to the trip to the hospital where, in the grips of the doctor's hands, they removed the unborn fetus from my womb. I fell off to sleep saying the Hail Mary . . .

Days passed into months and months into years. We tried to make the best of things but it became increasingly more difficult. The time was 1966 (during the decade of change) and Kelley was three years old. Women were beginning to assert their independence; that's what helped motivate me to leave Pierre. I was eager to assert my newly found independence.

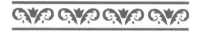

Chapter Four

Coming home to Huntingdon to live with my parents was not exactly my idea of asserting my independence or hardly a position they wanted to be in at that time of their lives. I had nowhere to go. I was not prepared to live on my own and support my daughter. Although I was grateful to have a place to stay, living there was suffocating. I did not have a life of my own. Things went smoothly enough until November 19, 1966 when a massive heart attack took my father's life while he was sleeping. The reality of his death took us all by surprise. He had had a prior heart attack, but did not appear to be in danger of another, since it had been five years since the first one. Needless to say, we were all devastated. It was a terrible time.

I loved my father very, very much. As a little girl all I wanted was my father's acceptance and approval. I wanted him to think I was the best, prettiest little girl and, like in the Hallmark cards that we all know about, I just wanted to sit on his lap, be hugged, read to and told how much he loved me. Unfortunately, that was not the case. I am not saying that my father did not love, even cherish, me but it was never spoken of. No one in those days was demonstrative with feelings. Your parents took care of you and that was the way they showed their love.

I will never forget the night just prior to my father's death. We were seated in the living room, my father in a chair reading and me lying on the couch feeling low and in a deep depression. My mother was in the kitchen preparing food. I started crying hysterically questioning my father as to why he did not love me. His heated reply was that he did love me, then he immediately changed it to the present tense saying, I do love you. The question that followed was one he could not answer: Why did you not show me?! Oh, how I wish I had never said those words. I know my father loved me, but at that time I was not so sure. My father's death so devastated me; it was so quick and painless and happened while he slept in the room just next to mine. I knew that night that something awful was happening, but as I lay there in my bed I became traumatized. Not wanting to think the unthinkable, I proceeded to ignore that an event just outside my bedroom door was going to result in the end of my relationship with my father. We had an unresolved issue and now there was no way to make it right.

Three months later, I earned the right to join the world again and make a life for my daughter and myself. Upon release from the hospital, I made the decision that my daughter and I must find a place of our own. I spent afternoons and weekends looking for just the right place. Places we saw were either in run-down neighborhoods, or if they were fairly nice, they were too expensive. We looked and looked until I finally found an apartment in Brentwoods that I could afford. We moved in immediately. It was special because it was our very first apartment.

Victor came into my life at a time when I was terribly vulnerable. I was in a time of need, both emotionally and financially. I met him while working as a temporary in a lighting plant on Long Island. He was a lighting engineer, intelligent, a man of color, personable, and neatly groomed. I liked him from the first time I saw him. I had a real need to please or I would never have allowed him to talk me into his horrible, evil world, to become a part of his insanity, but he did. He was not very nice; he used me for his own purposes. I should have known he was no good. I should have had more sense. He was a jailbird who used me to gain entry into the homes of upper-class communities on Long Island, picking my brains to find the areas of affluence. Maybe even pretending to love me.

The drive to Coram, New York took about one-half hour that beautiful, sunny day as the car sped along the Long Island Expressway. I put on the right-turn signal indicating that I would be exiting at Exit 50, North Ocean Avenue, heading north as the directions on the seat beside me instructed me to do. Kelley became very excited seeing the sign that read "Bald Hill" to the left at the top of the hill. The signs were marked "Ski Area," and Kelley's immediate response was "Oh, I can learn to ski." She was exuberant. That was not my plan. I had seen advertised in the local newspaper low to moderate rents for lovely one and two-bedroom apartments. I thought they might have something I could afford. That is where I was going when across from the sign that turned into Homestead Village was another sign that read "La Bonne Vie of Coram, NY." "Mom, look," Kelley yelled. "This is a great place! Let's live here!" I knew I would not be able to talk my way out of this one, so into the long flower and tree-lined driveway we went, facing a clubhouse with the huge letters spelling out the name of the complex.

Kelley so much wanted to live in the grand, gated-community, while I would have been satisfied to live across the street in a place not as grand, but one I could afford. Because of her seven-year-old determination, I was overruled in my choice, another step along the way of our journey.

Although everything seemed okay on the outside, there was turmoil in my inner world. My depression was still there and never seemed to leave me completely. To the world around me, I appeared to lead a normal life. I worked, brought up my daughter, dated with great effort. But I had no joy. Hidden in my inner recesses was pain. It was the kind of pain that never leaves. It wasn't physical pain, but emotional pain, scars from the past and unresolved issues. They were not intentional scars, but were scars nonetheless. My only comfort came from my dog, Artoo. He was my comfort. I could not tell Kelley or my mother about my tears. Neither would understand!

La Bonne Vie was a very lovely, newly constructed property sitting in the middle of Suffolk County, Long Island. It had villa-like architecture with cathedral ceilings and balconies overlooking thickly populated pine trees. We had a two-bedroom, spacious, modern, fully carpeted apartment with central air and a dishwasher. The best part was that Kelley and I had membership to the pool, sauna and tennis courts. Kelley made many new friends; she attended Longwood High School and did well preparing for her entrance into college. I made friends, too, but most of my time was spent on the road traveling to and from work. The rent was difficult to collect each month and I found myself having to make money in other ways. Through the years, these "other ways" have caused me a great deal of trauma.

I met Charles and Marilyn through one of my best friends. They were quite an unusual couple. He was a very distinguished, tall, black man with a handsome face and equally handsome features. He was striking as he walked into a room. His clothes were impeccable; they fit him to a T and were made of the best woolens money could buy. Some were even custom ordered. He really made an effort to look his best and was successful at it. He represented one of the finer furniture stores on Long Island as one of their top salesmen. He was quite the voracious talker and greeted everyone that entered the store with charm and personality. Everyone liked him. His wife, Marilyn, was an extremely tall, lean, white-skinned, dark-haired beauty from a very rich family on the north shore. She fell in love with Charles who had been sent to Long Island from Cleveland, Ohio to operate one of the furniture stores. She knew she was in love with him the minute she saw him. It was love at first sight. When I met them, they had recently bought a large house in the area and my friend and I went to see them and see the house. They had two beautiful children, a boy and a girl.

Charles began making eye contact with me from the beginning, even while his wife was in the room. I could detect that there was trouble brewing in their marriage. She would leave for weeks at a time, leaving the two children with her mother who lived nearby. Charles started calling me and when I would question him about Marilyn he would always say that she and the children were with her mother. He would ask me to come to the house or to go out to dinner with him because he was lonely. At first, I thought it was all right to do this, but after a while I could see a real interest growing. Before long, they each told me of their thoughts on separation and divorce. Given their situation, I was not totally surprised by this.

During this time, I was beginning to have real problems paying my monthly rent. The rent increase for the new lease period was an additional $70, which was more than my budget could handle. I did not know what I was going to do. So, one evening when Marilyn was at her mother's house with the children, I was telling Charles about it. He confessed to me that he and his wife were legally separated and that she would not be coming home. I displayed my shock at this news knowing that she often went to her mother's with the children, but I had not expected him to say that they had been legally separated for six weeks and that their marriage was over.

I struggled with paying the rent and kept getting further and further behind. I could not keep up with the increase in rent when Charles brought up the idea of Kelley and I moving into a part of the house that now had been vacated by his wife and children for a period of ten months. I could contribute to the household expenses and I would have a part of the house separated from him since the house was large. I jumped with excitement at the idea, knowing that Kelley would love living in this community in such a beautiful house, and knowing that I would be paying half the rent I was then paying. He was a friend, he and his wife had a legal separation, the house was large enough for us and I could save some money. It seemed like a plan, a very good plan. Little did I know that the situation was not going to work. Weeks later, I began to pack our things. Then, I received the news.

The phone was ringing off the hook. Picking it up, I said, "Hello?" I knew it was Charles. I silently listened as the news was being delivered over the wire of the phone that I held in my trembling hand. I was saying in the empty room, "What am I going to do now? I cannot afford the new rent." There was a long silence, it was deafening. "Where am I going to go? How could you do this to me?" Then, I slammed the phone down as hard as I could, putting an end to what I was hearing. We had no place to go. We had no home. My thoughts began to fly through my mind tripping over themselves in their haste. His call came while I was packing our things for the move. We could no longer move into his home. There would be countless repercussions for him in their divorce proceedings. I repeated this over and over. I could not get this out of my mind. Now what? One half of my possessions were already at his house. Where would I store my things? I thought to call Nathan, a neighbor in the complex only minutes away.

"Please, Nathan, help me. We have to leave my apartment tonight. I don't have the money to pay the increase in rent." A judgment was being served against me and my only option was the invitation to move in with Charles temporarily while Kelley finished high school and I found another apartment. But, now that was not going to happen. When Kelley came home from school at the regular time and saw Nathan with me, she knew something was very wrong. I was frightened to tell her that we would not be moving in with Charles as planned, that he had changed his mind, and that I had no money for the rent and that we had nowhere to live. Nathan brought a moving truck and packed all the furniture and food into it while I stashed the incidentals in the car. We had to find a place for Kelley to stay as I could not take her out of Longwood High School, since it was her last year, her senior year, and she was preparing for her admission to Harvard in the fall. I remember her being so angry with me, screaming abuses at me until Nathan finally calmed her down. With my car filled with all my possessions, and Kelley safely staying with the Marshalls, the parents of Kelley's best school friend, until we could make further plans, I headed to my mother's.

Kelley did well in school. She graduated with honors and, before I knew it, she was headed for Harvard. I felt we had made it. That was a point in my life where another decision had to be made. Kelley was off to college with her new life while I was left behind and still lurking in the darkness of a soul that had no joy.

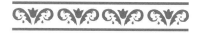

Chapter Five

It was a new decade, the start of a new life. It was 1980 when I met Mark. I now know that, like St. Mark, he was my guardian angel. We met at a time when we both were lost, lonely and vulnerable. Our meeting took place, not in a room where we dreamily looked at each other across a crowded room, but in the parking lot of a company where we both were employed. My life until that time had been filled with financial frustration, the agony of raising a teenager and the loneliness in which I lived. I was adrift in a sea of unworthiness and low self-esteem. Mark was a married man. He had been married too young to a woman he did not love but felt obligated to marry and remained married to out of obligation. He was there to rescue me and I to rescue him. We rescued each other.

His children, three boys, came soon after the marriage. When the third child was born, his wife decided her marital obligations were over. She had her boys. At the age of 31, he had been barred from the bedroom. They began sleeping in separate rooms. Feeling his rejection, he was looking for someone to restore his manhood. She was a good wife, but mostly she was a good mother. Mark and I found comfort in each other, but more than just a comforter he was my stabilizer in a time of conflict and fear. He was always ready and willing to give of himself. I would have been lost without him.

Then I met another lifesaver, a woman. She was recently divorced and needed additional income so she put her home up for rent. The house had a master bedroom, a private bath that overlooked a deck, a tree-filled yard and an Olympic-sized swimming pool.

I found the spiritual side of myself while I lived in this new place. I found my new church home around the corner. Finding my spirituality was my lifetime search. Through all the difficulties, God had always been there. His presence, His comforting grace, His light. Until the day I let Him into my life, I had never felt whole or complete. The moment I stepped into the little church around the corner and heard the choir singing, I knew I would never leave and that I'd never be the same. I had found my home.

That day was the first day of the rest of my life. I saw the light coming through the haze that was my life. I saw colors come alive for the first time; I noticed the small things that went unnoticed before. My hearing sharpened so that even nuances became loud and clear. Laughter felt like sunshine, tears flowed freely. Confidence, power and sociability were mine.

Kelley was in the university, money became less problematic and I had a new church home. Sitting in the back of the church for many years, I felt comfortable but detached. I would leave the church early, avoiding all traces of involvement. But slowly, over time, I began to participate in Bible study, seminars, the choir and other activities. I always loved to sing; I never professed to have a pleasant voice, but I sang anyway. My father always liked to sing. He would emote as if on stage performing some difficult song and he would get so involved. It used to make my mother and me laugh when he would begin to sing. He had a good voice, but I think he believed it was better than it was. I joined the choir at my church for the same reason: I loved to sing. Each week, we would practice on Mondays at 7:30 for one hour to prepare for the upcoming Christmas celebration. The day I was invited to join the inner circle of the church by the Naylors was the beginning of a new Christian life for me. They were my first church family, guiding me along the way with their love, actions and dedication. I was led to baptismal and membership into the church. Still in a minor state of depression, I managed my life quite well. I was still working, I was socializing and I had my involvement in the church. I was with God and I read my Bible. Still, the tugging at my heart was hard to ignore.

I started having doubts and fears about my relationship with Mark. The man who had been everything to me, sustaining me through times of financial difficulties, depression, helping with my relocation, being supportive in times of pressures with my work and with my daughter. He was a true friend. I believe he needed me as much as I needed him, just in different ways. Our symbiotic relationship convinced me that God had worked this all out for His purposes.

But I was becoming convicted of the error of my ways. I knew our behavior was adulterous and morally wrong. I tried to ignore the warnings. I closed my mind and told myself we were helping each other and that there was nothing wrong with that. Was that not what God wanted?

At last, I could no longer ignore the inner voice of God. I had to do something to make it right with Him. I had no idea the trauma and pain that would come from my decision to give up my good, dear friend by making it right with God. I had bound myself in a way and I had to let go. My sin was hurting me and hurting the One I loved. However,

31

Mark would not let go. He lost it one night when, in the middle of a heated battle, knowing that I was leaving him, anger built up inside of him. He became enraged. His face became red and taut; his eyes were on fire. He started calling me every name in the book. He cursed and swung my heavy Bible, throwing it in the middle of my glass-top dining room table, breaking it into shards of glass that scattered all over the floor. I was immobilized, frightened to death by his outrageous behavior. I could not move, I felt paralyzed with fear. Neither of us spoke for what seemed like an hour. The first words spoken were words of regret and promises of good behavior and a new glass tabletop. Words of forgiveness began tumbling out of his mouth in a rush that spilled over like a waterfall. He began making attempts to clean up the mess, asking me where I kept my vacuum and telling me not to come near the table so that I would not get any glass in my feet. I was so angry that I could not speak. I just watched him as he attempted to get every piece of glass off the floor and into the garbage.

Days went by, weeks, years. Mark had never gone completely from my life. At first, there was the harassment. He would call me at home, even ringing my doorbell until on two occasions, I called the police. When they arrived, they wrote their report and asked me if I wanted to have them make an arrest. Each time, after thinking awhile, I would say, "No." Then there were the phone calls on the job. We worked in the same facility. He could immediately connect himself to me by dialing the four numbers of my extension that separated us from each other. For years we talked by telephone, and on Christmas and my birthday he would send flowers. For years this was the relationship we had. He would call, we would talk, he would send flowers, I would politely thank him and on many occasions would share my bounty with the other girls in the office.

During this time, James came into my life. I had joined a very prestigious singles club that afforded me the chance to attend special events, dinner parties, theater and other activities especially planned for upper middle-class professional singles. We met at spots all over New York City to have a good time. I met James during that time. Our meeting helped in some way to give me an emotional attachment and we did have some fun together, but I learned very soon it was not to last. A newly-divorced man seeking adventure is not a sure bet for a long-lasting relationship.

I remember what happened to me at CFI, a small efficient business located in a newly constructed industrial park on Long Island. My job was in the records department and my responsibility was to keep accurate files on all the electronic parts for the company's inventory. Some of those parts were as small as my thumbnail. My desk was placed against a wall between two other desks. One belonged to Jerome and the other to Mary Anne. Both were in sales and their phones rang constantly and they'd have loud, forceful conversations trying hard to make a sale. I sat in that corner all day except for breaks and lunch. The pressure on these people was enormous and transferred to me somehow.

I will never forget the day when everything around me began to close in. I felt a darkness around me like the eye of a storm. Something was happening. I felt sick to my stomach, and then I heard the voices and ringing phones becoming softer and muffled. I began to cry and then scream out words I do not remember. All of a sudden, I felt the rush of people around me. Garrett Jean, the company CEO, was summoned. He rushed to my side. I felt his arm around me while he consoled and calmed me. All the employees were asked to leave the area for a few minutes. His warm words, calming my frazzled nerves, began to take hold and I began responding. He led me to his very spacious and comfortable windowed office where I could see the sun streaming in as we entered. Mr. Jean tilted the blinds to block the sun from intruding into the room. His calming words felt good. He encouraged me to deep breathe for relaxation and to imagine a place I would like to be right then. That was easy for me to do. I was transformed within minutes to another person who was visibly relaxed and controlled. My irrationality was gone and in its place was an inner and external peace. Mr. Jean instructed me to leave for the day and I did. The next day everything was normal. I sat at the same place and no one spoke about what had happened, trying hard not to broach the subject. And, things went on . . .

The day I came to ORT, March 5, 1979, I was nervous and had butterflies. I lacked the confidence I needed. I met everyone at a rapid pace; names were thrown at me and all I could do was say, "Nice to meet you." I was shown to my desk and left alone, for other tasks needed attention. Phones were ringing everywhere and when the phone rang on my desk, I froze. I didn't even know what to say.

I could tell from the beginning that I would not like Rosalie. She was Mr. McLaughlin's secretary and he was the director of the advanced developmental systems. I sat directly across from her while she sat directly in front of her boss' office. He would bark orders and questions at her that she would either answer or tell him she was waiting for the answer. Her typing was fast and accurate and she whipped the paper out of her IBM Selectric typewriter so fast that sometimes I thought it would tear. Rosalie could be on the phone making reservations at a hotel or airline, put them on hold while answering another phone or answering the questions that were posed to her at her desk. She was definitely a multi-tasker. She was pleasant, energetic, young, Italian and slightly plump. She was about 25 years of age with a good, high-spirited personality. Her mind was quick and operated at lightning speed. Orders were spilled out, while telephones rang at her desk. Her note taking and ability to hear and do many jobs at one time was impressive. I was impressed. Using her as my role model, I tried hard to type as fast as she did. Handling many jobs at once took a toll on me. Rosalie never helped me when I needed answers to questions regarding policy or the names of people in high places. All of this I had to figure out for myself. We did not get along well. I believe she sneered at my inability to type as well as she did. Maybe this was all in my mind, but I don't think so.

On March 11, 1991, the defense plant executed a huge layoff of 1,700 employees. We were not at all shocked by this news because, for a two-year period prior to that, some of our fellow employees had been let go. First to go were the CEOs and upper-management. Then an official "package" was offered to all the senior employees if they would retire early. Budget cuts followed. Promotions and salary increases were not forthcoming. Longer hours and heavier work-loads became the norm. Attitudes were poor and enthusiasm for our work was at its lowest level. When I was handed my paperwork and asked to clear out my desk, I could not have been happier. I immediately went to the restroom, entered a stall and began weeping and giving thanks to the Lord. He had answered my prayers. That workplace was not for me. It was never a comfortable place for me. My spirit could not tolerate the noise, ringing phones, clutter and confusion nor the pressure and stress. Even the florescent lighting and lack of fresh air and natural lighting were toxic to my state of being.

The day of the layoff was the beginning of a renewing of the relationship I had with Mark. His call came just before I was being escorted out of the defense building by one of the familiar guards I had known over 13 years and with whom I had developed a business friendship. Mark asked if he could take me home. I had no car at the time, but my cab was waiting so I declined his offer. When I had traveled the short distance home, there Mark sat in his car waiting for me. I did not know whether to be happy or angry. We talked for what seemed like forever. We ate together and then we decided to go straight to the unemployment office. That is how the renewal of our friendship began. It is a friendship that remains to this very day.

I quickly recovered from the layoff and Mark was hired, through a friend, to work at another defense plant.

I had to find work. My unemployment pay had lasted 26 months and now it was coming to an end. I had trained at the Long Island Business Institute where I learned computer and business techniques. The program at the school was called information processing. I did well with all the students in my class being given the award for best attendance and the student of the month award. I was extremely happy being awarded in that manner. Our course lasted three months and I decided to try to open my own business typing resumes, medical records, manuscripts, court records or just business letters. I purchased the equipment I needed and set up office in the small alcove in my apartment. I even invested in an ergonomically correct chair. Business went well, but there was not enough to pay the rising cost of living and so it all had to be dismantled, put up for resale, and I had to begin all over again.

Still unemployed, I put an ad in the laundry room offering to baby-sit. I was hoping one of the families at Summerset would see it and hire me. I waited but nothing happened. In the meantime, I had to get car insurance for the new car I had purchased from my retirement money. I chose State Farm because of their good rates and reputation. While I was making out the insurance paperwork, I started talking to Clarise, one of the agents at the local office. We became friends quickly and I told her of my need for a job. Once again, God was watching over me. She said they were looking for a file clerk for several days a week and that I should talk to Mr. Mann, the regional director. After doing this, I was hired to work three days a week. But before doing this, I got the baby-sitting job for Martin and Lisa. The baby's name was Rema and she was a handful. I never liked her. This baby was strong-willed, uncooperative, unloving and would not take a nap. She cried for everything and I know she didn't like me either. Finally, I started to resent her and became hostile towards her. Fortunately, Lisa became pregnant again, and she and her husband were buying a new home. So after nine months, she decided to stay home and I was able to leave that job.

Riding the bus one morning to class I met someone. Now, meeting someone on a bus can be a bit strange. His first approach was a look that turned my heart inside out, a look that penetrated my soul. I responded with a flash of my eyes that lingered on him for just the right amount of time, then quickly bounced toward the window. It did not stop there for I consciously looked at him again, the second time I was flirting and I knew it! When he moved from his seat to the front of the bus, my heart fell. I just knew he would get off at the next stop and I would never see him again. Instead he asked the bus driver for a transfer and started walking down the aisle taking the seat directly in front of me. He turned around and asked if he could sit next to me. "Yes!" I responded trying not to be too eager. Then the games began, the flirting. I was cautious, so it wasn't until after we had seen each other often on the bus that I would let him come to my house. He was good at flirting and also good at lying. I knew he was married but I chose to ignore all the signs. He used a beeper. I never had a number for his house and I never saw his house and we never met over the weekend. Those should have been enough clues, but I chose to ignore them. So, in December 1992, when he stopped calling and changed his beeper number, I knew, and it hurt.

Harringtons was my next port of call for a job. I read they were hiring for Christmas in a newspaper that was left in a cart at K&K in the parking lot. Something led me to take the paper and I immediately read the big ad for Christmas greeters at the store. I was hired as a door-greeter for the Christmas holidays and there I remained to become a sales associate nine months later. The store was in total disrepair, cluttered with too much merchandise, dirty bathrooms and kitchen, the flooring was never cleaned, the employees were rude, low-class and not the kind of people I would like to be associated with. The supervisors were no better, treating the people that worked for them with careless disrespect.

My first instinct was to leave that place and that bad neighborhood. One night at 9:30, I was leaving the store. I opened my car door, got behind the wheel, started the car and put it into drive, but my car was not moving. Upon getting out and careful inspection, I found that someone had lodged a huge box under the left rear wheel. I removed it by applying quite a bit of strength. Following that incident there were others, but I would not let that affect me. I kept praying for God's grace and kept handing out my spiritual tracts and even placing them in the coats that were being purchased. I never gave up on that and the hope that someday I would be out of that place. I made friends easily with my coworkers. The women I worked with each day were nice to me, but did not like the idea that Charlotte, my immediate supervisor, chose me over them to work in the fur coats department. She liked me in there for the way I worked with the customers, and gave them added attention and helpful conversation. But, even in there I could always slip a tract in the pocket of a coat that was heading out of the store to be purchased. I never stopped. Charlotte and Ted, our store supervisors, would, on many occasions, demand us to do something or to stop talking. I ignored it all. I kept the peace and continued getting the message out through my tracts. The place was seedy, but somehow I knew I belonged there for a while.

The day of the accident was a blur. I was out on the floor with the other women marking down coats on one of the high racks. We always complained about the shoddy equipment, the unsafe rolling racks that tipped over easily and were shoddily built. Their makeshift assemblies made them hazardous. We were between the tall coat racks, with our arms outstretched as we attempted to mark down the coats that were on sale. The rack gave way and all the heavy winter coats fell off the unattached rod that had been holding them. The pull of gravity made them fall quite rapidly. I tried to stop them from falling by holding the rack and trying to replace it in the grooves that had previously held it in place. What I remember mostly about this was the sharp pain I felt in my lower back and while experiencing this, one of my friends could not stop laughing. I screamed at her for her insensitivity and that is when it came to me that this was my way out of this place forever.

My life started a downward spiral. First there was the unbearable pain from the accident and then visits to chiropractors, neurologists, doctors, lawyers, hearings and court appearances. I had no money during this time. It never seemed to end. For two years, this was my life.

I immediately hired the law firm of Reid & Reid to represent me in a workman's compensation claim against Harringtons. I began seeing the chiropractor three times a week and the neurologist once a month. I had to make visits to strange doctors, those supplied by Harringtons, so they could examine me at length trying to unsubstantiate my claim for recovery and to make it null and void. But I pressed on. Finally, there were the court appearances with my lawyers and then with my doctors. Finally in 1995, I received my pension from ORT and the settlement from my accident. Following that, I received my disability benefits and Social Security Disability.

I thought I would never recover. Choosing Children and Family Health Center for my ultimate recovery was the best place for me. It started that day in intake with Inez who handled the interview before I could be placed with one of the therapists. My first formal meeting with Mr. Gordon began in August. He was a tall, slim, Jamaican man who made a practice of leaving his office to come out to the waiting room to invite his next client into his office. I liked that about him. He spoke gently, asking me to have a seat. I sat down in the cramped office. It was small and there were corrugated boxes everywhere, making it quite crowded. It did have a window and that was a blessing. Mr. Gordon was neatly dressed and clean but not a high-fashion dresser. He wore tweeds, shirts, and v-neck sweaters or vests. He spoke softly, pausing to allow me time to think and answer. Sometimes he said nothing.

I never missed a visit and he only missed two in a two-year period. I looked forward to seeing him and giving him a report on my success each week. As we talked, the "lights" would come on and I would become aware of my attitudes and behaviors and I constantly worked out ways to change the negative ones into positive ones. Everything became crystal clear as the minutes turned into hours, days, weeks and months. Time passed quickly. Matters and issues I had never examined came forth. I remember telling him of my fear of doing things I was not accustomed to doing, keeping everything in control and then one day I did something different. Instead of eating lunch in the familiar McDonald's, I went to Nathan's to eat. Another day I took a different route to go home and not the same old way. I had always been fearful of what was new or different. These might seem like small steps but they were a beginning.

Days spent in Mr. Gordon's small office transformed my life. I learned about myself and the more I learned, the more I longed to learn. Mr. Gordon was a good therapist. He lifted the veil from my eyes and let me discover myself. He revealed those things that had been hidden in my psyche. I worked hard to correct all my misconceptions about myself and Mr. Gordon helped me to do that.

Dr. Dormesy administered medicine to me once a month and followed up on my progress. Susan, the nurse, was exceptionally sweet and the staff became my friends.

During Christmas 1996, while attempting to send out Christmas cards to family and friends and decorate the apartment, something happened. I found myself in a disturbing mood. I was depressed—deeply depressed. Here it was, only eleven days before Christmas Eve, and I was suffering another despairing depression. I felt as if I would never recover. Why is this happening to me? What did I do in my life to deserve this? When am I going to get help? I was having a conversation with God. Please, I begged Him, help me to overcome this emptiness, this helplessness. Deliver me from this hopelessness, Oh God, please. I thought that I was having a breakdown.

Immediately, I called the office to talk to Mr. Gordon or Dr. Dormesy. Neither was there. Susan, the practicing nurse at the center, took the call. I was hyperventilating and practically screaming for the two men, my counselor or my doctor. She calmed me down in her very special way and when I was calm, she made a plan for me to be in touch with the doctor as soon as he came in. The day was endless. The hours crept by until, unable to stand it any longer, I made the call to him. I was later told that it was the best thing I could have done, because I was finally taking control of my life for the very first time. Speaking to the doctor he made the suggestion that I start taking the Paxil that he had first suggested on my initial meeting and evaluation visit with him. Not waiting for him to finish, I said, "Yes! Please put me on whatever you think might help." The prescription was phoned in to the local drugstore and I picked it up later that night. I have felt well ever since that night. I do not believe that it was the medicine totally. I believe in the grace of God who answered my prayer and that the medicine serves simply as an adjunct. My thanksgiving and gratitude belong to God who, in His infinite wisdom, quietly waited to hear me call out to Him for help. It was while in this state of complete agitation when I fell down on the floor and cried to Him for help, that I felt complete release from whatever it was binding me. The day this happened was December 13, 1996. Since that time, I cannot begin to tell the different ways my life has changed.

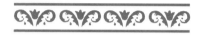

Book II – The Great Sin

"Give it to me, my dear. Give it to me. I will direct you in the way you should go. I know the plans I have for you, plans to prosper you and give you a good life." I heard this chant and these thoughts racing through my mind that drab gray morning. All I had to look forward to was my morning of meditation and yoga. Again I heard, "The steps of a good soul are ordered by the Lord. I can do things for you that you cannot do for yourself." Where were those words coming from?

I remember the first time I saw the light, the divine light, not the light of man, not created by man, not delivered to our homes by the electric company. No, this was different. I was in bed the night of the light. The room was completely darkened, there was no light coming in from a streetlamp, or a car's headlight coming through the bedroom window through the slatted blinds. No, this was different. My eyes were tightly closed and I began to feel a warmth come over me and then through my closed eyes I began to see a glow inside my mind. My mind brightened with light that I had never seen before. What was it? Where did it come from? The light became so bright that I was prompted to open my eyes to see where the light was coming from. I refused to do this, not believing that it was coming from some outside source, knowing in my heart that it was coming from within. I immediately knew that I was connected with the divine or the supernatural because it felt peaceful and serene. Then, it would slowly fade to black and it would be gone. No matter how hard I tried to bring it back, it could not be done. It happened again, this time while attending a service at church. For whatever reason, I have not had the experience lately. I do not know why but there are other ways that I know that the divine is in my life.

There was the morning of New Year's Day when I clearly heard a knock on the front door. I feared going downstairs due to the late hour, but I felt compelled to go to the door and open it. There was no one there, but I felt the presence that someone had been there. It was as it was when I was eight years old and kneeling by my bed. I always felt the presence of God in my room, so much so that I would invariably turn around to see who it was that was in the room with me. There was never anyone there, physically, but I knew in my heart that I was not alone.

Time and time again I have failed the test. He has been testing me and I still cannot seem to get it right. Why this struggle with good and evil? I am tormented by the adulterous relationship with my dear friend Mark. He remains married. It is a mortal sin being with this man who has been so good to me. If I am to follow the right path, following what the Bible says, I must turn from evil ways and repent and do what is right in the sight of God. Not doing so separates me from the love of God and His grace. Never being free from the attachment of sin, my life with Mark continues. That is when I keep hearing, "Give it to me, my dear, and I will take it and wash it and carry it as far as the east is from the west. It will no longer be your sin."

Julie, Mark's wife, never did anything wrong. She was a good wife and mother. The house was always fairly clean. The wash had gone through its cycle and was placed in the dryer. Later it would be neatly folded and placed in the appropriate places, ready for use by any member of the family. Meals were modest, prepared to specification. Julie stayed home; she was a housewife. She did not go out to a job or career, even after the children were grown. At times, she had a job working nights with an answering service where she alone handled the incoming calls for many doctors. She had her family, but no friends. She did not entertain and she was dedicated to her family. Julie had a problem; she was a recovering alcoholic and over the years gained much weight until she became obese. She refused to go to a doctor, although she had many physical problems. She would not leave the house due to her weight and other physical problems. This eventually led to her agoraphobia.

Reading was her pleasure until her eyes began to fail and they no longer allowed her to do the reading she so enjoyed. This luxury was no longer permitted. Fearing a diagnosis of cancer, she would not go to the doctor, even though her physical problems became more pronounced. Her parents died of cancer many years before and this was always her fear that the same diagnosis would someday be hers. She closed the door on her marriage after the birth of her third son so attempts at lovemaking for Mark were non-existent. Theirs became a marriage of convenience, remaining void of sexual desire, awkward and uninviting.

Her stroke came a few days before Easter. She fell from the bed that morning in a heap beside the night table. The sound was frightening and as Mark ran to the bed, he knew it would be disastrous. The paramedics arrived shortly, speedily taking her to the nearest hospital. Hours later, the doctor told Mark that his wife had suffered a stroke and would be paralyzed on her right side. Perhaps with therapy, she might regain some use of her arm and leg. But that never happened. Six years later, her condition remains the same. The wheelchair became her mode of transportation. The house was remodeled to accommodate the chair and Mark became her caregiver, turning his life over to take care of his wife.

I knew that he must be sent of God, this man who appeared to me while enjoying a few minutes before returning to work that October morning in 1980. I was more depressed than ever that day. I hated my job, the workplace and the people I had to deal with on a business level. But, there he was, someone that I was drawn to and he seemed to be drawn to me. He approached me carefully, not wanting to intrude. He told me his name and said he knew who I was and that I had only recently become employed by ORT. We spoke haltingly and then I remember him saying to me that he was married. I could have turned and run at that moment saying, "Nice to have talked to you," but I did not do that. Instead, I continued my conversation until it was time to return to work. He showed his gentleness when he placed his arm underneath mine and slowly guided me out of the way of a truck entering the parking lot. I liked that. I liked that a lot.

The first time he asked me to go out with him, I said, "Yes!" I could have politely refused, stating the fact that he was married. But, I did not. We went out to dinner, both of us obviously nervous about our dinner together, but when it was over, I quite boldly asked him if he would like to follow me to my home and that is how it all began that October in the year 1980.

Through many years of anguish, Mark was always there during the times when I felt unfit as a mother, having normal problems with my pre-teen and later, teenage daughter. It seemed many times that Kelley and I were in some kind of competition, me being a single mom and out in the singles world. There were the financial problems, not always being able to meet the high rent and pay the bills and keep my head above water. There was the insecurity about moving out of the field in which I was trained into another position I knew nothing about. I was promoted from secretary to buyer in the advanced development systems department and was relocated to the Grand Island facility to do a job that I was neither familiar with or knew anything about. Mark was encouraging me all the way. My pay and promotions from that time on were frequent, allowing me a better lifestyle for my daughter and myself.

On the downside, there were the times when I was quite bothered by this relationship. My affiliation with the church was growing, my faith increasing, and knowledge of the Bible was steadily growing to the point that I saw the evil of my ways by continuing this relationship with a married man. This was a mortal sin, one that God condemns, and I knew it. "Repent, repent," the words were always there. "Turn from your wicked ways and repent." I had now received baptism in water, joined the choir to sing at Christmas time and became a member of the church. And still I was bothered by my sin. There were thoughts I entertained, thoughts of going to New York City to live, thoughts of having him arrested for harassment, but none of these things could I do.

There were all the good times, too. We had fun together, enjoying each other in ways that cannot be explained. He treated me well, always remembering the great things as well as the small. He was gentle, kind and never a harsh word came out of his mouth. He treated me with such respect and always put me first. He could not do enough for me, even at the risk of his own and his family's welfare. I owed him a debt, I owed him something. I owed him a debt I could never repay.

Then, one night, it finally happened, that dreaded phone call in the middle of the night. You reach over to answer, knocking things out of the way in your frantic attempt to shut off the shattering phone in the middle of the night. You know it is something you do not want to hear and in spite of this, you answer. On the other end you hear a weakened voice that you recognize, but not like you even know the voice on the other end. It is quiet, whispered and sad. "Is that you, Mark?" It was. He began telling the story of his condition. That evening in his living room he felt the crushing, breathtaking, physically draining beginning of what he later learned was a heart attack. Asking his son to call the ambulance, he was transported to the nearest hospital only five minutes away. There he laid on a gurney in the crowded waiting room for over an hour before they attended to him. Then a team of emergency personnel made the initial diagnosis, which was not good. No one spoke as they went about their regular routine. After some time, he was told that he needed a quintuple bypass, a fairly regular procedure performed many times and at no real risk to the patient. "That was fine for them to say but this is me you are operating on," Mark thought and later related to me. He knew that the bypass was scheduled for the next morning. He knew he had to get in touch with me, for there was no other way that I would be informed as to what might have occurred. I said I would pray that everything would be all right and then I started praying the minute we hung up the phone.

Days passed slowly and I knew nothing of his condition. After a few days, I called the hospital, asked for his room number and was put through. I heard a man's voice, not Mark's, but his son's. I said that my husband and I were friends and worked together with his father and we were inquiring about his condition. He related that his father was out of the recovery room and appeared to be doing just fine.

That was the only way I could find out the information I needed to know. His father learned about the phone call later and knew that it was me who had called. Time went by and I finally got the phone call from Mark. What a relief it was to hear from him. Even though his condition was grave, it was still better knowing than not knowing.

His recovery took the prescribed six weeks and it was painful for both of us not seeing one another and not even being in touch by phone. In time, we went back to our regular Thursday afternoon lunch dates.

Things did not get any easier for Mark, still caring for his wife while in a precarious situation himself. I knew it was going to eventually wear him down. It took a lot out of him, taking care of Julie and now himself. There was the medication that had to be administered to Julie and then to himself. The taking of his blood and giving himself the insulin shots had to be performed each morning and night. The care and wrapping of legs each morning and uncovering them at night, bathing, feeding and all other household chores that had to be done. There were aids that would come in, but Julie was adamant about their arrival and did not want them trespassing into her home. That made it more difficult. Mark became her constant caregiver, leaving no life for him. He made it clear to her at one point that he needed one day away from home in order to do something for himself.

Once when I picked up the ringing phone, I heard Mark saying that he had to take Julie to the hospital the day before. She had fallen from the bed in the middle of the night and when he went to see what had happened, he found her crushed between the bed, the bedroom wall and the night table that stood by the bed. Obviously, she had attempted to get up to go to the bathroom and fell, crushing her face and hitting her head on the furniture. When he went into the room, she was covered with blood, clutching at the bed sheets moaning to him for help. Seeing her situation, he immediately called 911. Help arrived within ten minutes, the hospital being only a mile away. Six attendants, police officers and rescue personnel came in to take care of the situation. It took three men to lift her up from the floor and put her on the gurney, her weight being a great hindrance.

Mark felt so sorry for her. He knew her shame and embarrassment, as did I. A woman in that situation with six younger men in attendance, and your husband, all treating her with kindness and gentleness but her dignity was being shattered. Then her sons arrived having been called by Mark. He said he was going to the hospital to see how she was recuperating and then he said that he would get back to me with more information.

But then that night I dreamed of the headlines I had seen in the newspaper rack at the neighborhood gas station that morning, "Body Found—Brutally Murdered." The headline I could not forget. I stood there trying to read the story but my eyes could not focus on the names, addresses or dates, or even what had happened. The more I looked at the text, the more it became blurred. I blinked my eyes several times to moisten my lenses as the ophthalmologist had suggested, but it did no good. I searched in my pocketbook to see if I had another pair of glasses, but I had not brought them. Then a woman standing beside me said unhesitatingly, "What a shame, a man murdering his wife. What is the world coming to?" Before I had a chance to ask her any questions, she had walked away. I wanted to go after her and ask her to tell me more of the details, but then I became conscious that it would look strange, so I did not do it.

Not in my most vivid imagination could I have dreamed such a horrible conclusion to a life story that started out so innocently in Brooklyn, New York that year in February 1940. One night, in my horribly confused mind, I dreamed of a very dark, shadowy place. It was a place I did not know, a place I had never been or seen, but somewhere in my subconscious this place existed for me. Many times I visited this place in my dreams. One night the intensity of the dream was so overwhelming that I found myself on the floor having thrown myself out of the bed to get away from the horrors of the night. In this particular dream, there were headlines in a local newspaper: "Body Found—Brutally Murdered." The letters appeared larger than life. They appeared as large as news headlines for all to see. That is the way they appeared in my dream that night. I remember thinking that the body was found near where I currently lived and had been hidden in the scrub pines along the ponds and waterways. There was a large black bag used to cover the body and a huge cardboard box that contained the body. The dreams did not denote whether the body was male or female, its age or any other particulars, just a body.

I woke up that morning in quite a state. I was not able to fathom where such a dream would have come from or perhaps what it might be telling me. That entire day I was agitated and in despair over that dream. Sometimes, at night, I would be afraid to go to sleep, afraid I might have that same dream again.

Then one night it happened again. This time it was a man's body in that bag, in that cardboard box. I could not see his face and did not know who he was, but there was some kind of memory of this man in the black bag, in the cardboard box buried in the swamp area of the east end of Long Island. I didn't know who it could be or why I would be having this recurring dream. I felt this was just the beginning of a real nightmare.

The nightmares began when I learned that Mark was in the hospital the first time. In the past, I had never remembered my dreams. They were always bits of abstract pieces

that would float into my subconscious, would rattle around
for a while, until either finding a place to settle down or
move into another realm, leaving me feeling incomplete and
shaken. But this was different. These weren't jumbles of
thoughts or ideas, no spasmodic entering or exiting into my
space disturbing my sleep, no visual physical characteristics
or familiarity that I could identify. No, these dreams were
different.

Fire, a house burning. The house was near where I lived.
I knew that because there was a familiarity with the area. I
walk a lot and many times I will walk into town. I did this
often when I first moved to the east end of Long Island.
Learning about my new town was very important to me and
I enjoyed those long, solitary walks, making new discoveries,
stopping in the general store or the pet shop or even into the
Country Kitchen to have a bite to eat. *What a lovely town this
is,* I thought as I enjoyed a cup of steaming hot coffee and
watched the townspeople on the street scurrying around that
early fall day. But in the dream that night I saw a fire, a house
burning, a large black Hefty bag that was floating in the river
and the waterways that snaked their way through the east
end towns. Three hooded men entered my dream, not ordinary men but on the order of men out of a *Star Trek* film.
They kept trying to draw me close to them, but I would not
go. I saw a telephone on the ground, but the wire had been
cut. The phone had no attachment, just a lonely handset with
no connection. There were three cars in a gravel driveway.
They were old, abandoned cars, not having been used for
many years. They looked like cars from the fifties. The inte-
riors were torn and dirty, their exteriors were rusty, patched,
and had been painted again and again. They had flat tires like
four pancakes that seemed to be melted into the ground.

Voices surrounded me, but were unfamiliar, as if they were speaking another language. I felt helpless as these people continued trying to draw me nearer.

Other dreams were similar but included one where I had been declared legally blind. I had trouble accepting that fact as I moved from place to place in slow motion, stumbling over everything in my path. Colors came to me in bright hues, but there were also the shadows that gave me the feeling of helplessness. The only bright spot was that with the fading of my eyesight, my other senses, hearing and smell, were accelerated. The smell of kerosene was acute in my nostrils, the orange-red of the fire was like dragon tongues, wrapping around everything in sight. I found myself moving across the bed in a vertical manner as if to get away from the licking flames. Someone was smoking and was blamed for the fire in the house. There was also a body brought out from the fire and that is when I woke up.

One dream caused me to flip out of bed. I found myself on the floor and the lamp stand had been knocked over. The haze over me was not from the fire, but from those people who were smoking drugs. What exactly they were smoking, I did not know, but I did recognize the odor. I started calling for someone to help me and then I saw a hospital bed. Mark was in the bed but the sheet had been pulled over covering him from head to foot. How I knew it was him, I do not know, but I knew. I felt myself asking, *Who is going to help me now? Who will be there for me? Now, I am completely alone. There is no one. I don't have Mark, so I have nothing. When did he die? Why didn't I know about it? How would I know? There is no one to tell me. I do not exist in his life. We have a secret life.*

In my dreams there were always police officers, firemen and rescue workers. Constantly present were these same people always asking questions, making notes and rushing around frantically. Firefighters often pedaled bicycles or scooters. It was as if a circus were in town. In this dream, there was a hangman's noose and men throwing knives at a revolving target to which a man was tethered and the wheel was spinning. Unicyclists were running into each other. There were colored balloons that were huge and were flying high and were being burst because of the planes in the sky that were shooting at them. Everywhere there was noise, not music but noise. Blaring sounds that had neither melody nor rhythm were accosting my ears. Confusion abounded, nothing was normal, colors were too bright, the people were weird. I didn't know what I was doing there or who I was. That same feeling was in my mind as I opened my eyes that morning.

Mark was not feeling well. He had not been feeling well for a long time now. The day we celebrated my birthday at one of the finer restaurants in the area, I made a commitment to him to always be friends no matter what happened or did not happen. He said that he had waited to hear me say that for 21 years. I knew at that time that it was not a good day for him. Would I see him again? I did not know. The following Thursday, our usual day to be together, he did not call and I did not see him. For four days I heard nothing. I started trying to trace his steps. I thought about the local hospital. I went there to see if his car might be in the parking lot. He was known to drive himself to the hospital on many occasions. This was not the case that day. I found the street on which he lived and tried to locate his car, but to no avail. I just waited and prayed. That was all I could do. I called the hospital to see if he had been admitted, but they were not able to give me that information. I looked his name up in the phone book to find a telephone number. I found his son's. As the phone rang, I panicked. I started to hang up but when I heard the message I went further leaving my name and tele-phone number and asking to be called. I did not hear from him, so I waited.

There was a winding path taking me and my companion deep into the swallowing riverbed covered with strong old oak trees. The deeper into this place we went, the more fear-ful I became. My companion said nothing. Then the cell phone rang and the conversation between the driver and the other person on the end of the phone was tacit, short with no actual conversation. I knew this was not good. *Why did I ever get in this car? Where are we going?* Again, I woke up before I could find the answers to the questions.

Julie, Mark's wife had her stroke just before Easter Sunday in 1996 and that changed their lives completely. Her diagnosis was complete paralysis on the right side of her body. Her overweight condition, having been an alcoholic most of her adult life, and the onset of diabetes did not make her condition easy to deal with. Her weight had grown to almost 300 pounds, which was putting a strain on her heart. Her weight made it difficult for her to move. She was a smoker with high blood pressure, which condition she neglected because of her refusal to take the medicine ordered by her doctor. Her eyes began to deteriorate preventing her from doing the one thing she really loved: reading. Her limbs swelled to three times their normal size and that put an added burden to her already unhealthy body. She would never go out, not even into the backyard to see the fauna and flora that her husband was so fond of and planted to make the yard pretty for her. The birds had their own individual hotels handmade by Mark and were hung in the trees and on the fence that separated their home from others on the street. She did not talk to anyone on the street, preferring to be left alone. She neither spoke to the neighbors, nor did her family visit. Even her sons seemed to stay away from the house, only visiting occasionally out of obligation.

The house they lived in was built in the early sixties, one of many in a community of moderate priced houses for those moving to the east end of Long Island. These small Cape Cod houses were built on small parcels of land with attached garages. They lined the streets for miles. The houses had no basements and were built directly on slabs of concrete. They cost approximately $10,000 to $16,000 and were swallowed up by working class couples that were moving out from the city to the suburbs. Raising a family in this environment was the perfect place for young people. Mark worked at a defense plant, one of numerous plants on Long Island. Before this job, there was the aluminum siding business, but a salesman he was not. ORT, in the crib—a place where electronic parts were inventoried—was his first job of many. He was young, only 27, married and with three boys. He had to make a living for his new family. He traveled 33 miles in each direction to and from work, which was fine in the beginning before the traffic built after many years and many people made their exodus, leaving the city for the suburbs.

He did well in his job, working overtime and never taking a day off. Through the years, he was moved out of the crib and given responsible jobs in the program management department. He was not comfortable in some of these positions due to the stress and politics of the workplace. That was where I met him and that was how we began our lives together.

After Julie's stroke, things really changed in the household. His sons were married and moved away and that left Mark and Julie together. The house had to be retrofitted in order to accommodate the wheelchair. Medical assistants and aids started coming in three times a week to attend to Julie. Over the years, this care had to be discharged due to the expenses that were accruing. Mark became the only caregiver; he did everything for Julie. He was a dedicated husband taking care of her every need without complaint. The only bright spot in his life were his weekly Thursday visits to see me.

We continued to see each other through the years, even after Julie's stroke. It may have been only twice a week and sometimes not even that much. But, we still stayed in touch. Our relationship moved from employees working together, then dating and finally to a higher level of closeness, intimacy, sharing of everything. We were confidants, lovers and best friends. We were well-connected, soul mates, right from the beginning.

The three hooded men were in my dreams again. Out of the mist, I saw them slowly approaching me. I wanted to run, but something kept my feet rooted and grounded so that I could not move. They were shrouded in a liquid mist that almost completely hid them except for their heads that I could see but not distinguish. It's not so much that they appeared mean looking, because they did not, but they were menacing. One of the men reached out his crooked finger and beckoned me to come closer. I felt stuck, as I did in my life, I also felt stuck in my dream. What did they want from me? I heard the one say something about the harvest being ready but the laborers being few. What does that mean? Is that something I heard in my Bible study class? What are they trying to say? Before I could figure it all out, I began to see something flying high above them like big black birds, maybe bats or something bigger. I searched the sky to try to determine what it was but I could not. The men seemed to know what it was and looked up to see as if they were awaiting their coming. But when the planes came closer, they began to fall from the sky one after another landing not far from where we were standing. Planes were falling from the sky. *What is happening?* I thought. The planes never crashed to the ground, they merely fell, gliding their way down to earth, settling softly one by one. *Planes falling from the sky,* I repeated to myself. *What does it all mean?* People began to exit the plane. They were all well and healthy and appeared to be relieved that they were here in this place. What is this all about? I wanted to ask the three men, but was afraid.

The three hooded men went to greet the new arrivals. There were about 27 in all, men, women and children of different ethnic backgrounds and all seemingly very happy with seeing the three hooded men and I, still deathly afraid of it all.

The water was overcoming me; it was surging like a great tidal wave. We had heard that there may be tidal waves on Long Island at some time, but was this it? The water was higher than the rooftops. You could barely see the tops of the many trees. I felt, as the wave washed over the house I was in, that this was like the mighty Holy Spirit baptizing me like they did that Sunday evening in late March of 1985. First, there was my testimony, and in front of all those people who were my church friends but still strangers, I started with, "I am no longer mine but Thine." I could see them all looking straight at me with nary a smile on their faces. I ended with, "May this covenant made on earth be ratified in heaven, Amen." That was it. That said it all. The pastor, deacon and myself moved slowly down the steps of the baptismal pool and when all was ready, the blessings having been said, my head being held and my nose closed, they gently submerged me under the water and lifted me quickly again. I remember that night so well. So why am I dreaming this particular dream? Do the huge waves represent the submergence of everything to be blessed by the Holy Spirit? I wonder. I wake up startled and cannot go back to sleep for the dream. The dream won't let me. I had questions with no answers.

The dreams continued.

"Drive the car, Vicky," he yelled, "drive, I said." When I started to move, I saw the open car door and Bobby's leg was half in and half out of the car as it was speeding away from the curbing. "Oh, hell," he yelled. "Well, you told me to move." I realized that we were heading for the hospital. The sirens were blaring and all the cars on the street swerved out of the way of this careening car as we moved quickly through the city. Upon arrival, there were nurses waiting and a staff of attendants that quickly went about the business of attending to the patient. The patient was comatose, I heard, and his vital signs (it was a man) were weak. I did not, at that time, realize that the patient was Mark. "Is he going to die?" I asked. "No, he is not going to die, but he will never be with you."

"Let me go, please, let go of me! You couldn't put Julie in a home. You can't do that to her? Well, what about me." We argued for a long time. "Your son will think bad of you. Well, maybe my daughter thinks bad about me all these years being with you, a married man. But, what about my feelings? You have a family. I want my Christian family. I do not want to be left behind because of sin. I don't want eternal damnation. Do you?"

The dream came from my desire to run away from the whole situation. The dark hooded man slowly approaching me with his finger pointing to me, wanting me to step forward was the beginning of God's calling. I was afraid and wanted nothing to do with this stranger who wanted me to join him. His voice was soft and gentle but his look was ominous. He called unto me. His words echoed in my head and heart as he said again, "The harvest is full but the laborers are few." I wanted to join him, but still I resisted.

There was rain and snow on the day I went to the Criminal Court Building in Riverside, New York, and my only hope was that a verdict would be brought in before the snow covered the roads and made them unsafe for travel. When I reached the parking lot of the building, there was complete gridlock. There was no place to park. I drove a ways from the main building and had to walk quite a distance before I entered the building. Security was there in full force and as I emptied my pockets and made my way through the security check, my thoughts were on Room #11 where the Honorable George Cory would render his decision. I hurried to the room, past the guard sitting at the table outside the swinging doors. My footsteps could be heard echoing, their sound like pennies failing from someone's pocket on the bare tiled floors. The silence was deep. I opened the doors and as I entered all eyes were on me, including the newspaperman I had talked with the day before while waiting for the jury to return to the courtroom.

It was 12:00 when the jury finally came in. Each juror giving his "Yes!" to the question as to whether they all agreed with the decision and then the verdict was given. The verdict was guilty. That is when I woke up, because the man in the chair who had just been sentenced to 50 years in prison was Mark. I suffered through the pain of that dream as if it were real. The snow was failing harder than it had been before I entered the building and I made my way back to my car.

Then, there were no more dreams. The dreams previously dreamed became reality.

Crossing the busy parking lot that snowy winter morning, I thought about those incredibly moving dreams I had had in the past. I could not get them out of my mind. I was so engrossed at one point, that I did not see the approaching car on my left. Even though his headlights would certainly have been a warning, I did not see them. I passed the service station on my way to the courthouse where, in my dreams, the gasoline had been purchased and used to burn the house down after the murder. It still frightens me every time I see that place. I won't even buy my gas there even though it would be convenient for me.

Once I entered the courthouse and went through security, I looked for a public telephone to call my friend and relate to him the latest update on the case. He would ask me questions and I would answer to the best of my ability.

I entered through the courtroom door as I had done in the dream, but this time it was real. This time it was not one of my horrific dreams. The jury was out deliberating and there was another case being tried in the interim. The courtroom was not as crowded as it had been in my dream, but the deafening silence was the same. Serious faces I saw all around me, everyone cloaked in heavy winter clothes, scarves and hats that had not even been removed. They all sat like robots, no one saying a word, afraid to break the silence that permeated the room. Maybe they thought if they spoke, they would miss something important. When the jury returned with their solemn but determined faces, I knew the news would not be good.

The twelve sat down, each with their own sad face, as if they were tired and heavy-burdened with the issues and concerns of this trial. I searched these faces, one at a time. Twelve strangers there to determine the life of one person, someone they did not even know, someone whose life and surrounding lives would be changed forever.

The accused, handcuffed, was again brought back into the room and allowed to sit down next to his attorney. I saw in these faces the devastating news that would come in a very few minutes. I prepared myself for the obvious. I prepared myself for the inevitable, sitting stiffly in my chair, afraid to breathe, holding my breath and not blinking an eye. The stony faces, one by one, delivered their guilty verdict when asked by the judge. After what seemed like hours, the sentence was delivered. I thought I would faint. The air in the room became heavy, my throat closed and my eyes were unfocused. I trembled with fear. The judge then announced the charges. Mark faced 25 years to life in prison on the murder charge and up to another 25 years on the second-degree arson charge at his sentencing, which was scheduled several months in the future.

Then, and only then, could I look at him. His eyes were like blue pools of water. His hair, usually neatly groomed did not seem so on this day. Even his mustache had not been trimmed and his face was unshaven. I could not continue to look at him. He looked at me with a death stare. I tried to wave my hand and smile a little but could not pull it off. It would not have looked right. I did not see any of his family there and he had no friends except me, and I was glad that I was there for him. I could not believe what was happening. His life was shot, just like that. Was it disillusionment with his life? Was it the fact that he had to be a caregiver for the rest of his life or was it that he could not be with the one he truly loved? I will never know. I heard him say, "I love you," as the armed guards removed him from the room.

Will I see him again? Probably not. He was a huge part of my life. You cannot forget someone just because they become sick. I will never forget him. I pray for him each and every day. Maybe one day I will see him in my dreams, but until then I can never forget.

I know I will not hear from him again. My whole world, those around me and my very inner being have all been affected. I could not receive calls from him, nor did I really want them.

After that, I dedicated my life to God and His amazing grace. Life does have meaning. People have a special place in my life. There is meaning and a hope that I never experienced before. I don't see things in the same old way. Everyone has noticed the changes in me. There are those who have been close to me that see the difference. Those who have known me casually could not see the pain beneath the mask. They knew nothing of the pain I carried around each and every day, the pain that never went away. It walked with me; it was with me while I was wearing my forced smile. It was the tears behind the smile, leaving me when I slept, but there it would be to greet me in the morning hours. How do you get away from yourself and your thoughts? How do you fight the enemy within when you do not know that enemy?

Well, I learned that the enemy was me. I was that enemy fighting against myself. I felt invisible, stagnating in a pool of self-loathing and negativity. Once I realized this, I could help myself. Mr. Gordon was the one who made me see who I was, my potential, and what I had to offer the world around me. Thank you, Mr. Gordon.

Although medications have become my constant companions and relieve the depression and anxiety, it is me who has changed by the grace and mercy of God. I am a better me, a wiser, loving, giving human being. God will never stop changing me and molding me in His image. That is what life is. It is not the destination but the journey to become what God has purposed in your life.

Life centers, for me, around my relationship with God, others' problems and concerns. I now have the compassion to create a loving atmosphere around others in order to make their lives better, more productive, meaningful and happier.

About the Author

Victoria Heirston graduated from John Adams High School and Pace University in New York City. She is divorced with one grown daughter.

Before retiring, Ms. Heirston worked for the defense industry on Long Island for over 27 years. In addition, she does volunteer work with Literacy Volunteers of America.

Victoria enjoys reading, classical music, fine restaurants, the theater, and traveling. She also loves long walks on the beach, gardening and solitude.